Promoting health through primary health care nursing

A guide to

quality indicators

for commissioners

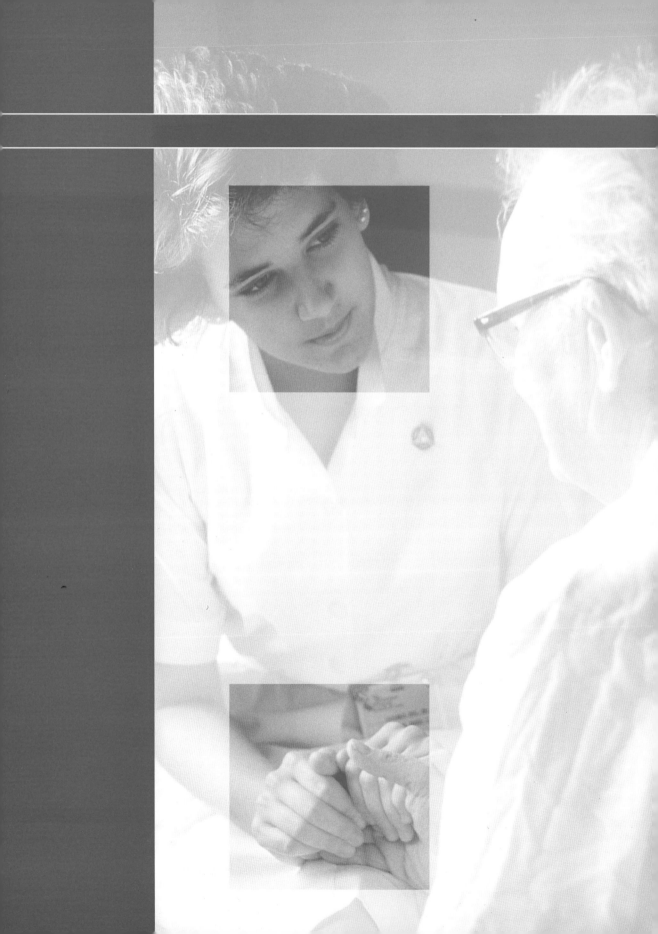

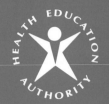

Promoting health through primary health care nursing

A guide to

quality indicators

for commissioners

Acknowledgements

The research project team from King's College, London comprised Jill Macleod Clark, Sue Latter, Jill Maben and Helen Franks. The HEA project team were Bernie Evans, Anju Bhabuta, Amanda Killoran, Jean Spray with assistance from Anthony Morgan, Hilary Whent, Karen Ford and Briony Enser.

The project was supported by a number of key professional advisors who made a valuable contribution to the project and to the development of the guide. The HEA and Nightingale Institute gratefully acknowledge the input from: Nickie Bainbridge, Lambeth Community Care (NHS) Trust; Norma Brown, Optimum (NHS) Trust; Liz David, Ravensbourne (NHS) Trust; Noreen Day; Amelia Eystom, Wandsworth Community (NHS) Trust and Sheeylar Macey.

We are indebted to the many clients who contributed to the project by providing a consumer perspective. We are also grateful to the colleagues who commented on the drafts of this guide and to the many commissioners, clinicians and health promotion professionals who shared their expertise and knowledge. A comprehensive list of all such contributors can be found in the main project report entitled *HEA's developing quality indicators project* (HEA 1997).

ISBN 0 7521 0943 X
© Health Education Authority, 1997
First published 1997

Health Education Authority
Hamilton House
Mabledon Place
London WC1H 9TX
Designed by Persona Grata
Printed in Great Britain

Contents

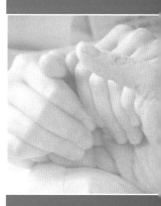

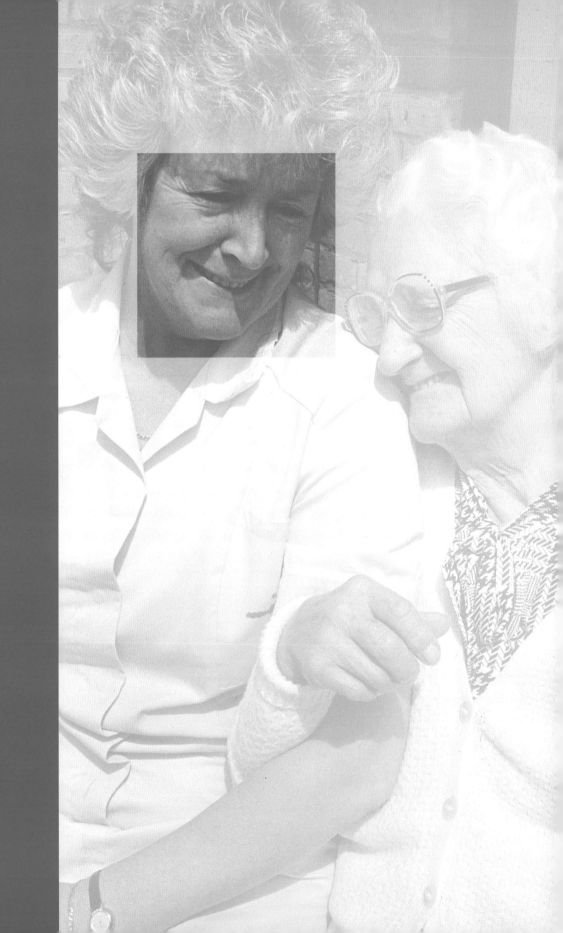

Foreword

The Health Education Authority has produced these guidelines in response to demands placed on primary health care nursing services to enhance the commissioning, delivery and evaluation of their work. They were developed over a two-year period within which there have been a number of changes in health policy, and an increasing emphasis on demonstrating quality in the delivery of health care.

Further changes in policy and terminology are now inevitable with the renewed interest in and concern for public health. These changes will bring with them a continuing need to identify ways of demonstrating and measuring quality. However, mechanisms and indicators for assessing, measuring and setting quality standards remain scarce. This is possibly a reflection of the preoccupation with the quantitative measures of outcomes and targets, as well as the undoubted challenges of developing robust quality and process indicators.

These guidelines demonstrate that it is possible to identify and measure quality in the process of primary health care nursing interventions. They also illustrate the links between quality in the process of interactions between the client and the primary care nurse and health gain. The guidelines are firmly rooted in research and practice, and offer a valuable starting point for commissioners and providers to introduce better quality assessments into the commissioning process.

The need to demonstrate quality and value for money in primary health care nursing has never been greater. We hope that these guidelines will act as a stimulus and incentive for commissioners and providers to work in partnership to meet the challenge and to build on the framework of quality indicators, standards and mechanisms to reflect local priorities and needs.

Jean Spray
Director

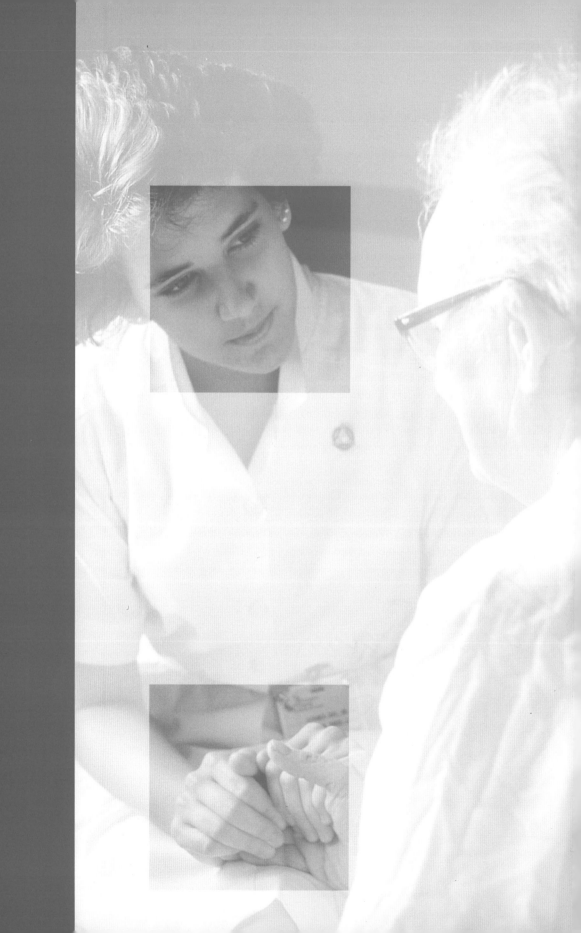

Introduction

Purpose of the guide

This guide has been developed from the findings of a research project commissioned by the Health Education Authority (HEA). The aim of the project was to explore ways of measuring quality and effectiveness in the health promotion work of primary health care nurses[1,2] and to identify indicators of quality which relate to effectiveness/health gain/positive health outcomes.

The findings from the project provide an evidence-based framework for commissioning primary health care nursing services. This framework can be used to inform commissioning and purchasing and achieve maximum health benefits for clients.[3,4]

The purpose of the guide is to support these processes by:

- illustrating the link between quality in nurse–client interactions and potential health benefits and outcomes;
- demonstrating the importance of focusing on quality when commissioning services designed to promote health;
- providing a framework for measuring effectiveness in primary health care nursing services through the use of process indicators to determine potential effectiveness;
- identifying factors in the primary health care setting which inhibit and facilitate quality and effectiveness;
- suggesting ways of auditing and monitoring indicators of quality and health gain in primary health care nursing.

Whilst the guide has been designed primarily for commissioners of PHC nursing services it is also relevant to PHC nurses, NHS Trust chief executives and to directors of primary care nursing services within Trusts. It attempts to clarify issues of quality and effectiveness in PHC nursing by highlighting the relationship between quality in nursing services and positive health outcomes. These are relatively uncharted waters and the guide represents some early steps in the demanding process of trying to locate, understand and ultimately measure the concept of quality in this area of nursing.

The context

Managing for quality is a key objective of the National Health Service (NHS). This is outlined in *The National Health Service – a service with ambitions* (DoH 1996a, pp. 44–5), which states that, 'Ultimately, it is those who provide the service direct to patients who can determine the quality of care, and they have a special role in developing quality standards, assuring quality and auditing their own performance. People working in health authorities also have an important contribution to make, in creating the conditions and providing the stimulus for a quality service.' The document further underlines the commitment of the NHS to provide high-quality care through an 'integrated health service which is organised and run around the health needs of individual patients, rather than the convenience of the system or institution'.

Quality in health promotion refers to the structure and processes underpinning a nurse-client interaction leading to health benefit. These are described by Donabedin (1992) as comprising of technical care and the interpersonal attributes employed by nurses to implement them including: effectiveness, efficiency, acceptability, legitimacy and equity.

3. It is acknowledged that use of the term 'client' rather than 'patient' may be controversial. However, the term 'client' has been used throughout this handbook to denote patients, customers or users of PHC services. The term client is also used in recognition that many people accessing the service are 'well' and do not necessarily require medical treatment for ill health or disease.

4. The terms 'commissioning' and 'purchasing' are often used interchangeably. The two terms do however differ in meaning in that purchasing concerns the exchange of contracts and money whilst commissioning is more concerned with the strategic planning of services of which purchasing/ contracting is only one part.

The emergence of consumerism and the development of patient charters provide fundamental underpinnings to the evaluation and monitoring of service delivery and evaluation (Ross and Mackenzie 1996). In *Primary care: the future* (DoH 1996b) five principles of good quality primary care are highlighted. They are: quality, fairness, accessibility, responsiveness, efficiency. The present government's forthcoming national health strategy *Our Healthier Nation* (updated version of the *Health of the Nation* document) and Green Paper on public health will further reinforce these principles.

The *Health of the Nation* White Paper (DoH 1992) set goals and targets in health promotion and disease prevention in line with the World Health Organization's *Targets for Health for All* strategies (WHO 1985) and the WHO draft document *Health for all for the 21st century* focuses strongly on the role of the PHC nurse. PHC nurses will play a key health promotion role in developing health services in the future working collaboratively with other agencies and professionals. The contribution of nurses, midwives and health visitors to good health promotion practice and attainment of *Health of the Nation* targets (DoH 1993) clearly defined that:

- Nursing practice should be evidence-based.
- Clear objectives and targets consistent with *Health of the Nation* targets should be set.
- Environments for health care delivery should be conducive to achieving the objectives.
- Nurses should have clear responsibilities and authority for health promotion.

It is therefore crucial to identify and evaluate the role of the PHC nurse in influencing health gains. In order to achieve this objective it is essential to make the activities of a PHC nurse much more explicit and to measure the impact of such activities. To date there has been no appropriate framework or model for informing the commissioning and monitoring of PHC nursing interventions. This guide provides the starting point for this important process.

Methods used to develop the indicators

This guide is based on the research findings from a study of PHC nursing practice. An initial set of indicators of quality and effectiveness was generated which could be linked to positive health benefits for client groups. A focus group approach was adopted to gain professional consensus using accident prevention strategies as the model. Further consultation then took place with a wider audience of clients, purchasers and providers, and the remit was broadened to encompass a range of health promoting activities undertaken by PHC nurses. Particular attention was paid to clients' perceptions of quality and their descriptions of the health benefits of PHC nursing interventions. The relevance and validity of the initial set of quality indicators was tested in practice through a series of in-depth case-studies of PHC nursing practice. As a result of this process, key process indicators of quality were identified and these form the basis of the guide. The empirical data demonstrate how these indicators link with tangible measures of effectiveness in terms of health benefits and intermediate health gains for clients and longer-term health outcomes and targets.

The collaborative case-study research involved extensive participant observation and interviews with all stakeholders including health authorities (HAs) and GPs (fundholding and non-fundholding), provider managers, PHC nurses and clients. Further data were collected via tape recorded and transcribed nurse-client interactions and tape recorded in-depth interviews with clients. An outline of the research project is presented in Appendix 1 (*see* p. 31). Full details of the research can be found in the project report *HEA's developing quality indicators project* available from the Health Education Authority (HEA 1997).

Structure of the guide

The material in this guide is presented in five main sections.

- ○ Section one examines the need to focus attention on issues of quality in the process and outcome in PHC nursing interventions.
- ○ Section two defines ten process indicators of quality in nurse–patient interaction which emerged from the underpinning research and demonstrates how these indicators lead to health benefits.
- ○ Section three provides a checklist of the prerequisites for achieving quality in PHC nurse interventions and highlights what should be looked for when commissioning for quality.
- ○ Section four addresses quality in practice through the presentation of real life case scenarios and examines the process through which health benefits are achieved.
- ○ Section five provides a quality framework for performance management through audit.

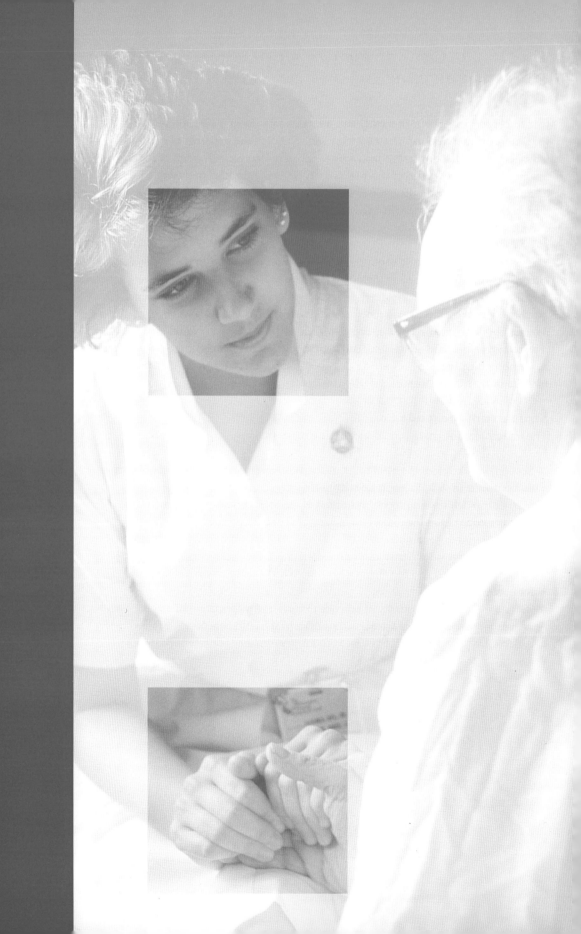

The need to focus on quality in primary health care nursing

The large number of PHC nurses[5] in the United Kingdom represents a huge resource for enhancing the health of the population. This resource must be fully utilised. The promotion of health and preventive health care is fundamental to the role of PHC nursing for clients, families and communities and it often supports people at critical times in their lives such as childbirth and old age. The potential for nurses to play a major role in helping individuals and communities to lead healthier active life-styles is immense.

There is growing evidence that nursing interventions can lead to significant health benefits (Imperial Cancer Research Fund OXCHECK Study Group 1994, Family Heart Study Group 1994). The value of nurse-led health promotion clinics and risk awareness programmes has been clearly demonstrated (Laidman 1987, Gibbins *et al.* 1993). However at present, performance indicators for PHC nursing services tend to focus almost exclusively on quantity rather than quality or measurable health benefits. PHC nursing is generally assessed using the Körner data collection system and similar methods which simply provide a numerical indicator of the number of visits made or contacts achieved (Crown 1996, Cowley 1996). Other approaches to quality management have been adopted, e.g. Qualpacs, Monitor and Senior Monitor (Kitson *et al.* 1988), but these were not designed for PHC settings and again focus on efficiency rather than effectiveness and have been, in the main, hospital-based tools.

The focus on achieving a maximum number of contacts clearly influences the way that PHC nurses work. There is constant pressure to demonstrate effectiveness and efficiency through maintaining or increasing the number of contacts. Such an approach is counter-productive as it masks the real health promotion purpose of PHC nursing interventions and ignores issues of quality.

Until recently purchasing for health promotion has largely been influenced by *The Health of the Nation* (DoH 1992) targets and measured through longer-term bio-medical outcomes. These fail to take full account of the short- and medium-term behavioural and social changes which can also be put into effect (Brown and Piper 1997). This is not to say that quantitative measures have no value but rather that in PHC nursing they are self-limiting and will only provide information about the number of client contacts rather than illuminate a wider spectrum of health outcomes. The importance of process in HP interventions and the need to achieve quality in nurse–client interactions at both individual and community levels is increasingly recognised (Ross and Mackenzie 1996).

Commissioners and providers are currently seeking more meaningful ways of examining and defining nursing practice (Griffiths 1995, King 1995). While the measurement of quality is in its infancy there are a number of innovative approaches and tools which can be used, for example the organisational audit tool used by the King's Fund (1996).

Recent Department of Health initiatives and White Papers emphasise the need to explore and expand roles in PHC nursing and midwifery (DoH 1993, 1996a). A

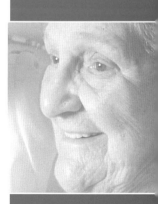

5. *It is estimated that there are approximately 45,000 qualified nurses working in the PHC sector.*

1

recent *Executive Letter* (DoH 1996c) encourages new approaches to effectiveness and supports the development of quality indicators. It also endorses contracting mechanisms which are innovative, especially those that utilise client perceptions of effectiveness.

Shifting the focus of contracted activity and outcome measurement towards process and quality presents a real challenge. The research which underpins this guide has confirmed the view (Donabedin 1992, Dahl 1995) that a key determinant of quality in the process of promoting health and delivering health care is the interaction between the client and the PHC nurses. The nature of the nurse–client interaction appears to have a fundamental influence on whether or not the client derives health benefits from such contact. This guide offers some descriptors of a quality nurse–client interaction which will lead to improvements in health. The prerequisites within a primary care setting for facilitating the delivery of quality interactions are also identified. Examples from the case-studies are used throughout to demonstrate the impact of such interactions on health benefits.

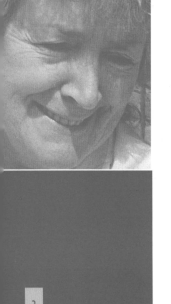

Ten indicators of quality in nurse-client interactions

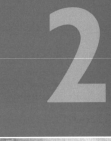

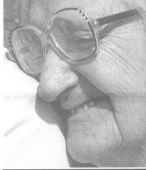

The nurse–client interaction lies at the heart of PHC nursing practice and the ten indicators of quality[6] which emerged from the research both describe the characteristics of an effective nurse–client interaction and offer a framework for evaluating the quality of such interactions.

There is clear evidence that the extent to which these characteristics are present influences the achievement of health benefits. They therefore offer a framework for predicting and measuring effectiveness in terms of short-, medium- and long-term health gain. In practice the indicators rarely appear in isolation and effective interactions will be characterised by several of these indicators.

The ten indicators of quality in PHC nursing

1	**Choice of services and accessibility of service to client**
2	**Sufficient time**
3	**Skilled assessment of health needs**
4	**Informed and credible practitioner**
5	**Individualised approach**
6	**Client-centred partnership approach**
7	**Non-judgmental approach**
8	**Continuity of care**
9	**Acting as an advocate for the client**
10	**Liaison and collaboration with other professionals and agencies**

The ten indicators emerged consistently from interviews with clients and observation by the researchers in the PHC setting. They represent what is seen as important by clients and what clients believe make a difference to them in terms of health benefits, confirming findings from other quality and outcome studies (Redfern and Norman 1994). Diagrammatic representation of the way in which the indicators of quality impact on health benefits for clients can be found in Appendix 2 (*see* p. 32).

Each of the indicators has the potential to be used to inform commissioning decisions about PHC nursing and more specifically they can provide the basis for meaningful systematic evaluation and audit.

Examples are given of how each of the indicators can be identified in practice and how this impacts on health benefits. The examples are illustrated with quotes from the research participants and, where possible, with reference to other empirical work. Suggested audit routes for the measurement and monitoring quality indicators are also outlined.

6. A quality health indicator is a marker of aspects (or characteristics) of quality which improve health outcomes. Barić and Barić (1995, p. 152) describe indicators as: 'variables, which can be used to design or to measure the success or failure of a programme'. Indicators of quality link the process of a nurse–client interaction with the structure necessary for them to take place and the benefits or health gains which result.

CHOICE OF SERVICES AND ACCESSIBILITY OF SERVICE TO THE CLIENT

The client view

"I know how to get hold of the nurses quickly; I can pop into the clinic or phone them."

The evidence base

The time and place of interactions between nurses and clients is seen as critical by clients in determining the effectiveness of the interaction (Luker 1990, Roberts *et al.* 1996a). Clients and client groups need to be able to access PHC nurses at times of need. Requirements of a nursing intervention are continually changing and PHC nursing services need to be flexible to optimise client benefit. Issues such as locality, equity of access, approachability and timing of the services are key components of this indicator. The elderly client quoted above had multiple health problems including hypertension and angina. His anxiety levels were reduced markedly by feeling he had easy access to the nurse. Whilst it is impracticable to meet all 'felt' client needs, priority groups and communities must be targeted and service delivery should be flexible and responsive to change.

The nursing perspective

"Clients need nurses 24 hours a day. This means making services such as clinics responsive to the needs of the population and reviewing them regularly. Sometimes a home visit in the clients own environment can be the best place to get to the root of a problem or meet a need more quickly at other times they can come to the clinic."

Suggested audit routes

- Client feedback on perception of access, flexibility, approachability and timing of contact, e.g. surveys using methods such as interviews and questionnaires.
- Audit of nursing service information available to clients
- Audit of uptake of services to identify poorly used clinics and other facilities.
- Audit for flexibility and ease of access to the service.
- Audit of client satisfaction with the care received and their perceptions of resulting health gain.

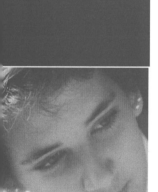

The client view
"I didn't feel rushed but comfortable to bring up what I needed to say."

The evidence base
Good listening skills were identified by clients as critical to nurses understanding their health needs. An important factor in being able to do this was that the PHC nurse must have sufficient time (Macleod Clark *et al.* 1992). During the project, clients expressed appreciation of the opportunity to talk about their health needs. Getting to the root of the problem or health need can take time but is more effective and efficient in the long term because client needs will be identified and health gain will result. In the case-studies it emerged that when the PHC nurse had the opportunity to listen to and understand the main health needs of clients and families, both clients and PHC nurses perceived that health needs were addressed promptly (Dahl 1995). For example one health visitor, who took time to listen to local mothers, recognised that maternal isolation was a problem. The health visitor then organised a parent and baby group where parents had the time and opportunity to support each other with advice and support from the health visitor.

The nursing perspective
"Sometimes getting to the bottom of a problem takes time. It's much better to give this time, especially initially, because then the real needs are identified rather than wasting time with non-issues or not identifying a health need at all."

Suggested audit routes
- ☺ Monitor for evidence of balanced skill/grade mix to give the PHC nurse time to work with clients and to enable appropriately trained, registered specialist PHC nurses to be responsible for needs assessment, care planning, evaluation and review of client health status.
- ☺ PHC nurse feedback of ability to give time to clients.
- ☺ Client feedback on whether they feel that they have enough time with the PHC nurse.

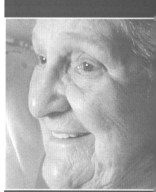

SKILLED ASSESSMENT OF HEALTH NEEDS

The client view

"The health visitor ran a low cost accident equipment scheme and pointed out the possible danger of my children falling from the window. I hadn't thought about it before but she helped me to make the windows secure."

The evidence base

The importance of accurate assessment to identify health needs has been well documented (e.g. Summers and McKeown 1996). In the above example the PHC nurse carefully and sensitively assessed the risks and was able to make an accurate judgement of health need. The PHC nurse then devised an evidence-based plan of actions which were acceptable to the client (as advocated by McMurray 1992). By drawing on her knowledge of the local and national prevalence of childhood accidents the health visitor was able to identify the risk to the children in the home environment having previously set up a low cost accident equipment purchasing scheme. Accurate assessment of client health needs is frequently multifaceted and changeable. It is important to note that this indicator is concerned only in part with the use of nursing 'assessment tools', it is also concerned with actively listening to the client's expressed need and incorporating elements of the other indicators identified by this research project.

The nursing perspective

"I bring my own experience and expertise as well as the research and guidelines that we work to. I think that this is what makes best practice and increases the chances of health gain."

Suggested audit routes

⊙ Client feedback on perceptions of benefits, health gains and changes in care/behaviour patterns subsequent to PHC nurse assessment and intervention.

⊙ Scrutinise health needs assessments/profiles to determine that assessment and identification of local health need has been made.

⊙ Audit professional development strategy and skills assessment development.

⊙ Audit of client-held records to demonstrate documented PHC nurses' goals for health benefits and evaluation of its effectiveness.

⊙ Audit and evaluate the uptake and outcomes of schemes such as the one in the example above e.g. uptake of equipment loaned to clients and evaluation of setting up a low cost loan scheme.

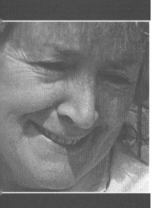

The client view

"The nurse knew a lot about asthma. I didn't think that I could control my asthma but the nurse really showed me that it could happen. I cannot really say that I have asthma now because I haven't had an attack in over two years since I first went to her, before that it was awful."

The evidence base

The effectiveness of nurse–client interventions is influenced by the extent to which the client perceives the health professional to be knowledgeable and credible (Macleod Clark *et al.* 1992). Credibility in the eyes of clients arises from them recognising that PHC nurses have acquired expertise and use their knowledge, skills and experience to help them to understand and manage health problems. The client in the example above required frequent hospital admissions prior to having her illness managed by a skilled practice nurse. Working to guidelines and protocols, the nurse taught her to monitor her breathing and take appropriate action to prevent asthma attacks from occurring. This client moved from a position of 'ill health' to gain understanding and control of her asthma and was subsequently able to return to work. She continues to visit the nurse to review her treatment although her visits are now less frequent.

The nursing perspective

"When a client believes in your advice and sees that what you said actually works they'll believe you more readily the next time."

Suggested audit routes

- Client feedback on the value of advice and information and PHC nurses' credibility.
- Monitor for appropriate skill/grade mix and resource allocation e.g. a named PHC nurse who manages care for a client/client group.
- Audit of care programme approach by PHC nurse e.g. managing clients with asthma.
- Audit of access to training and updates e.g. on management of asthma.
- Audit process and achievement of academic and professional development for key PHC nursing personnel.

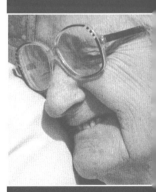

**INDIVIDUALISED
APPROACH**

The client view

"The nurse takes an interest in me, she helped me think about losing weight but understood that I will always want to eat some of my favourite foods. She talked through my likes and dislikes and we looked at my diet and adapted the plan to suit me. I've lost the weight and kept it off."

The evidence base

Clients are individuals and care needs to be assessed and planned in terms of the client's individual circumstances and perceptions of need. Quality care planning must be both supportive and non-prescriptive to enable the client to achieve maximum health gain. Further evidence of the importance and value of individualised care can be found in Twaddle *et al.* (1993) who demonstrated how individualised support can lead to a decrease in the number of contacts required by clients.

In the above example the nurse based the care plan on the client's own circumstances. She worked individually with the client, who was diabetic and overweight but who also wanted to continue to eat her favourite Caribbean food. By doing this she supported the client to continue eating preferred foods whilst helping her to reduce her weight and eat a healthier diet.

The nursing perspective

"Getting to know the client individually is very important. The advice and support that you give can be of more practical value and you can build on that."

Suggested audit routes

- ○ Audit client perspectives of the extent of individualised care and care planning.
- ○ Audit client records for evidence of HP goal setting and individualised assessment and planning.
- ○ Monitor consistency of content of training programmes in order to meet local health needs.

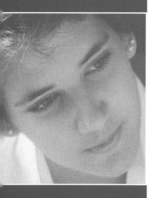

The client view

"I really wanted to stop feeling so low all the time, the health visitor recognised this and helped me to get better."

The evidence base

Client viewpoints, priorities and goals must be given precedence in care planning and delivery. Setting agendas and health goals important to the client and in partnership with the PHC nurse, is imperative in delivering care that is perceived by the clients to be both relevant and supportive to them. PHC nurses have a role in helping clients to make these decisions, based on the clients having the full knowledge and information which will enable them to make rational choices. Identification of the priorities most important to achieve their own health goals enables the nurse to target care to areas most relevant to the client and thus most likely to be taken up and maintained by the client. Therefore health issues that are most important to the client should form the focus of the interaction and should be identified by the client. There are links between this indicator and indicators three and five which denote the need for both an individual approach and one which utilises effective interpersonal skills (such as listening to the client's own definitions of need) in the context of a skilled assessment (for examples see Rourke 1991, Timpka *et al.* 1996). Understanding behaviour change techniques and recognising a client's readiness to change, enables PHC nurses to educate and support clients through the different stages of change as part of a planned programme. This is critical where nurses aim to achieve long-term improvements in a client's health. The example highlighted above showed that the health visitor worked through issues using skills and expertise with the client, supporting her when she experienced postnatal depression.

The nursing perspective

"Starting from the client's own beliefs means that you can use your knowledge to support them to make changes and achieve what they need to."

Suggested audit routes

- Client perceptions of whether their priorities and preferred approach is used can help them achieve health improvement.
- Audit of client records to determine evidence that the client was involved in goal setting and action plans, plus the outcome of the care plan.

CLIENT-CENTRED PARTNERSHIP APPROACH

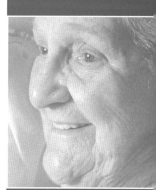

**NON-JUDGMENTAL
APPROACH**

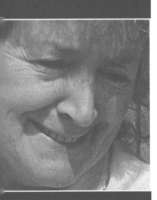

The client view
*"I am going to make my own decisions. I wasn't being
criticised for my own beliefs, that made me feel more secure
with the nurse."*

The evidence base
Value judgements by nurses, without heed to individual client views on their health,
and without considering the social, environmental and political influences which affect
people's abilities to change, can lead to a 'victim blaming' approach (Latter *et al.* 1992,
Dines and Cribb 1993). One client described how she was very anxious that she would
be judged to be a 'bad parent' because she had not been able to fully implement the
sleep management plan that she and the health visitor had agreed to. The PHC nurse
spent time allowing the client to talk about her problems, as well as listening and
making suggestions rather than telling her what she must do. As a result of this the
client started to feel more confident and less anxious, knowing that she could set her
own achievable objectives to move towards her goals at her own pace. The next week
when she returned for a further appointment she said that she had made marked
progress and felt very good about her ability to make change happen.

Where attitudes and behaviour change are imposed by practitioners, i.e. an expert-led
'top down' approach, clients become the subject of an intervention rather than an
active participant in health change and treatment decisions.

The nursing perspective
*"Blaming people for unhealthy behaviours only alienates them
and they think 'Well I won't go back there'. That gets you
nowhere in the long run. It's better to help them to make
changes at their pace and give them the information and
support to help them to make up their own minds."*

Suggested audit routes
⊙ Client feedback on perceptions of whether a non-judgmental approach is used to
   support them.
⊙ Monitor training availability and attendance e.g. for communication,
   interpersonal skills and behaviour change techniques, as well as including 'equal
   opportunity' training and race and cultural awareness.
⊙ Audit to show that the client record demonstrates that both the client and PHC
   nurse have set realistic and individual goals to achieve desired outcomes.

The client view

"I can see the same nurses. This means that I know that they know me and I know them which makes it easier to ask about things even if I think it might be a silly question."

The evidence base

The evidence for encouraging continuity of care is compelling (Savage 1995). Clients in this study found it beneficial to be able to see the same PHC nurse or nursing team over a period of time. Trusting relationships develop where partnerships between clients and nurses are formed. For example this parent who had a sustained relationship with the health visiting team telephoned them when she was worried about their child's health to ask for advice rather than making an appointment to see the family's GP. Clients said that they preferred to talk to nurses who knew their personal and medical history rather than have to explain their circumstances to new people every visit.

The nursing perspective

"Working in a team means that we can offer a more continuous service and someone is usually available to assist clients most of the time. They [the clients] get to know us and trust the service when they see how it works for them. The service is long term and sustained leading to less dependence and more individualised care."

Suggested audit routes

- Client feedback of perceptions of continuity of nursing care and its health benefits.
- Scrutiny of client-held records to demonstrate that the client has access to nurses they are familiar with.
- Audit evidence that each client has a 'named PHC nurse' i.e. a qualified registered nurse who undertakes assessment and care planning.

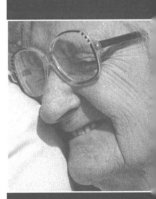

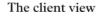

ACTING AS AN ADVOCATE FOR THE CLIENT

The client view
"The asthma nurse said that she'd talk to my GP about changing the asthma treatment for my daughter. It was a great relief, I felt that I would sound like I'm complaining, but they work together."

The evidence base
The importance of advocacy to achieve health benefits has also been emphasised in work by Appleby (1991) and Gillespie (1996). The PHC nurse may often act on behalf of clients and families to represent their views and needs. In the above example the nurse recognised that the parent needed support and representation of the child's needs in order to use the GP service effectively and efficiently. The child's medication was altered as a result and the child subsequently experienced less severe symptoms of asthma. This indicator also encompasses the important public health role of PHC nurses in their role of raising awareness of health needs at both local and national policy levels.

The nursing perspective
"I see my role not only as being a hands-on nurse but also as negotiating for clients at an organisational and political level."

Suggested audit routes
- Client feedback of their awareness that PHC nurse has acted on their behalf.
- Scrutiny of client records for evidence that advocacy has occurred where appropriate.
- PHC nurse feedback to elicit evidence of the ability to appropriately advocate for clients and client groups, and of other co-ordinated public health activities.
- Audit multiprofessional working practice in PHC and evaluate its effectiveness.

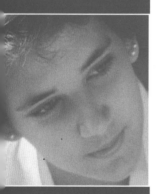

The client view

"The nurse put me in touch with someone who had a special understanding of my sarcoid condition."

The evidence base

Communicating and co-operating with other specialist professional groups and agencies maximises efficient use of resources and minimises professional duplication of services (Kendrick 1994). The practice nurse in this example put the client in touch with a local sarcoid group to enable the client to talk about her own personal fears to others with the same problems. The client subsequently reflected that she felt more positive and relaxed about the disease and how she would cope.

Individual and community health needs should be addressed by the multidisciplinary team (MDT). One way of achieving this is through meetings where team members have the opportunity to discuss individual cases and plan care and service developments. At a public health level the MDT can work together by profiling the health needs of the practice population and developing strategies to meet the health goals, for example, by participating in activities such as the annual 'No Smoking Day'.

The nursing perspective

"We [the PHC team] organised a health promotion day. Nurses, doctors and therapists from all community groups were represented. It was a great success and we reached lots of people. There was a lot of follow-up afterwards for the nursing and medical teams. It really felt as if we were raising awareness of health issues and the services available."

Suggested audit routes

- Complete an annual health profile for the locality.
- Monitor the frequency of MDT meetings at which action points are recorded.
- Client feedback to elicit the benefits of MDT shared care.
- Audit for evidence of interagency collaboration and interprofessional working practices.
- Audit client nursing/medical records to identify instances of duplication within the team.
- PHC nurse feedback of problems encountered (if any) with liaison and collaboration with other professional groups and agencies.
- Monitor that MDT training and staff joint training and development opportunities are available.

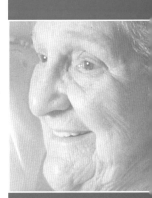

3

Prerequisites for achieving quality primary health care nursing interactions: a checklist

However well motivated an individual nursing practitioner may be, their success in delivering a high quality and effective service will be determined in part by the organisational infrastructure in which they work. The research highlighted the influence that certain features of PHC can have on a nurse's ability to deliver quality interventions. The most important variables centred around physical environment, management structures, and organisational culture. Frequently identified barriers quoted by the participants included high caseloads with a need to focus on crisis intervention; the absence of clear preventive health-led strategies; and the requirement to meet contact-led rather than needs-led targets. Other reported barriers include emphasis on long-term rather than shorter-term outcome measures; fragmented team structures with poor liaison; and lack of opportunity to develop a flexible and innovative service to meet clients' health needs.

It is possible to define a set of standards or prerequisites for an infrastructure required to support the PHC team, which will facilitate the type of nursing interventions that can achieve health gains. The responsibility for ensuring these prerequisites are in place rests with both the provider manager and the commissioner. The provider manager has a day-to-day remit for ensuring quality services but they may only be assured if the comissioners explicitly demand these standards within written service agreements. Those GPs who are currently fundholders have a dual responsibility as both a purchaser and a provider of services. If such standards are stipulated in the contract requirements set by commissioners, they can also provide the basis for measuring and auditing of quality.

The essential prerequisites of a PHC system which enable PHC nurses to incorporate quality into their working practices at both individual and public health levels are outlined in the Table opposite.

The checklist of prerequisite features outlined opposite highlights areas that should be looked for when commissioning quality PHC nursing services. It provides a framework for predicting the extent to which the quality indicators are likely to be in place and poses questions which commissioners might ask to ensure that prerequisites are being met.

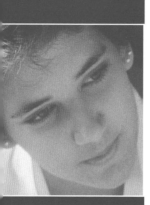

Explicit HP goals and strategies for PHC nursing interactions

- Are goals explicitly stated and are they embedded in principles of preventive care?
- Are goals articulated in terms of the achievement of measurable short-, medium- and long-term health benefits?
- Do goals and strategies move beyond crisis management, the achievement of contact targets and national policy outcomes? (Brown and Piper 1997, Buck *et al.* 1997)

Partnership approach

- Do clients hold their own records?
- Are clients involved in defining their own health goals and making decisions?
- Are clients involved in service needs identification and evaluation processes?

Appropriate skill mix

- Does the skill/grade mix provide adequate numbers of highly skilled PHC nurses to undertake adequate assessment and complex interventions? (Jeffreys *et al.* 1995, Cowley 1993)
- Is the skill/grade appropriate to meet the health needs of the population?
- Are support staff trained to an appropriate level?

Integrated team work

- Does the MDT demonstrate clear structures and roles, MDT care planning, communication mechanisms and collaborative networks and information technology systems such as e-mail? (King's Fund 1996, Ross and MacKenzie 1996, Antrobus and Brown 1997)

Appropriate environment and flexibility

- Is there choice in terms of venue and out-of-hours services for PHC nursing input including home- and community-based visiting depending on client need?
- Is the clinic environment user-friendly and accessible to all groups of consumers? (King's Fund 1996, Roberts *et al.* 1996b)

Profile of health needs

- Are PHC nursing-planned interactions defined by locally identified population health needs profiling? (Peckham and Spanton 1994, Billings and Cowley 1995, Summers and McKeown 1996)
- Are shared databases utilised to ensure collaboration and reduce duplication? (Ross and MacKenzie 1996)

Appropriate evaluation strategy

- Are providers using a range of audit and measurement tools to evaluate the quality of their services? (Mant and Hicks 1996, King's Fund 1996)

Practice development strategy

- Are providers demonstrating active investment in PHC nursing staff through access to further education, libraries and current research?
- Does this include skills updating and specialist training?
- Are practice guidelines and protocols continually updated to reflect new research evidence? (Antrobus and Brown 1996, 1997)

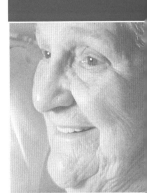

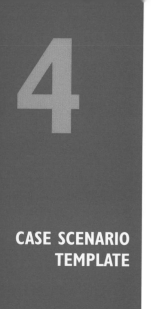

4

CASE SCENARIO TEMPLATE

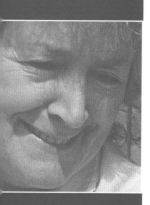

Quality in practice – case scenarios

The data collected during the case-study research provides some graphic illustrations of the important relationship between quality nurse–client interactions and the resulting health benefits. The general principles which lead to health gain and the links between the ten indicators of quality and the processes which result in health gain are shown diagrammatically in Appendix 2 (*see* p. 32). A series of scenarios are presented in the next section to show how specific and measurable improvements in health resulted from the presence of quality indicators and how specific features within the primary care setting supported delivery of quality services. In each scenario the link between health benefits, quality interactions and the features of PHC setting is presented using the template illustrated below.

Health gain for client
- Tangible improvements in health status, well-being and quality of life.
- Coping, adapting and changes in knowledge or behaviour pertinent to health status.

Quality health interactions with PHC nurse
- The influence of the ten process indicators on quality interactions.

Goals and actions of PHC nurses
- Promotion of physical, cognitive, social and educational development.
- Empowerment of clients, families and communities to prevent disease and minimise existing ill health.
- Enable individuals and communities to adapt and cope with life events.
- Eliminate or reduce the underlying causes of disease rather than treating the resulting ill health.
- Reduce the impact of ill health.
- Arrest or retard the progress of chronic health problems.
- Compensating for the effects of life events.
- Prevent avoidable accidents/incidents.
- Identify delayed physical, cognitive or social milestones.
- Impact on *The Health of the Nation* (DoH 1992) targets by identification of individual, environmental and local causes of disease and ill health to maximise potential for health and well-being.

Prerequisites
- The structural and organisational elements which give the opportunity for quality characteristics to be incorporated into PHC nursing practice.

Auditing measuring and monitoring quality
- The purchasing and auditing framework which drives the process.

Adapted from Ishmael and Duffy (1995).

The following scenarios have been extracted from real life examples of nurse–client interactions. They demonstrate the link between the quality process indicators, the prerequisites and the resulting health benefits. Although these scenarios are specific examples from the project case-studies they offer generalisable principles which can be incorporated into any PHC nurse interaction with any client group.

Supporting a family with asthmatic children

In this example two children had been diagnosed with asthma. Their mother was very anxious and did not know much about the disease. The practice nurse advised her about how to manage, control and prevent the symptoms. The mother then decided to stop smoking in the home. The practice nurse taught her how to use the asthma inhalers effectively and communicated important information to the family health visitor, school nurse and GP. The school personnel were also advised and supported to manage the symptoms of asthma.

Health gain for clients

Children with asthma not exposed to tobacco smoke.
Children's asthma controlled and managed at school and home.
Target: *The Health of the Nation* Coronary Heart Disease (DoH 1992).

Quality health interactions with PHC nurse

A mother's experiences

- *"I was able to see the nurse at the clinic that day to get advice."* (Indicator 1)
- *"I was so shocked and needed a lot of time to talk about asthma."* (Indicator 2)
- *"She told me what I needed to know to help my children like not smoking in the flat."* (Indicator 3)
- *"I trust her because what she's told me has helped."* (Indicator 4)
- *"The nurse knows that these flats we live in are damp and not ideal for asthmatics."* (Indicator 5)
- *"She took into account how we live."* (Indicator 6)
- *"I wasn't told not to smoke any more but how I could help my children to avoid the smoke."* (Indicator 7)
- *"I can pop in and see her whenever I need more advice."* (Indicator 8)
- *"The nurse talked to the health visitor about my housing."* (Indicator 9)
- *"The nurse gave me leaflets to take to the school so that they would understand."* (Indicator 10)

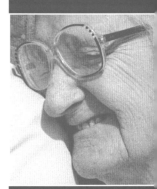

Goals and actions of PHC nurses

- *Promotion* of children's development by giving the parents and school personnel information about asthma and preventing associated complications of asthma. Liaison with and working in partnership with the school nurse.
- *Empowerment* of family to prevent asthma attacks and minimise asthma symptoms.
- *Enable* the family to cope with and manage asthma symptoms and the mother to achieve a change in smoking behaviour (Stretcher *et al.* 1993, self-efficacy; Gillis 1995, mother changes behaviour).
- *Eliminate or reduce* the children's exposure to tobacco smoke.
- *Reduce* the impact of the diagnosis and problems associated with asthma on the family.
- *Arrest or retard* the likelihood of acute and chronic asthma symptoms.
- *Compensate* for the potential health implications of having asthma by increasing awareness in the family of how to manage the disease.
- *Prevent* avoidable asthma attacks and symptoms.
- *Identify* delays in physical, cognitive, social and/or educational development associated with asthma through effective disease assessment and management.
- *Impact* on *Health of the Nation* Coronary Heart Disease targets (DoH 1992) i.e. smoking behaviour.

Prerequisites

- The PHC nurse is able to work to explicit goals using strategies with outcomes which are measurable in the short, medium and long term. The PHC nurse also works to locally agreed strategies to achieve health behaviour changes.
- Appropriate skill/grade mix support to the PHC nurse so that they can use skills and expertise with the client.
- The PHC nurse is a member of the MDT and communicates effectively with other members of staff and other agencies.
- The clinic environment is user-friendly offering an open access clinic.
- The PHC nurse has access to practice data which shows the prevalence of asthma in the local area and has appropriate knowledge of asthma.
- The client case-notes and client feedback enable evaluation of the effectiveness of treatment to take place.
- The PHC nurse is trained and regularly updated in asthma research and care.

Auditing, measuring and monitoring quality

- Client feedback to confirm ease of accessibility to the PHC nurse in times of need, that the nurse was approachable and that there was sufficient time with the PHC nurse. Client evaluation of the extent to which they were involved in goal setting and treatment planning. Was the care client-centred and non-judgmental? Feedback from the PHC nurse regarding the above and ability of the PHC nurse to work in a health promoting way.

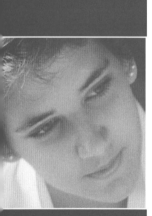

- Client feedback concerning their perception of the efficacy of the advice and information given to the client.
- Audit the client-held and nursing/medical records for evidence of the stability of the children's asthma. Has the mother sustained her health behaviour change? Documentation of interagency collaboration/communication with the school, health visitor, school nurse and hospital accident and emergency departments.
- Audit the type of support staff available and what their roles are within the PHC team in relation to the overall service delivery.
- Audit that the PHC nurse works to evidence-based and up-to-date protocols and guidelines.
- Count the number of clients seen during the clinic and the time taken with clients and compare it to other times and annual numerical returns.
- Does the practice have a chronic disease register?
- Check when the service is used most heavily.
- Audit the nature of client visits and contrast them to known local and national health needs.
- Audit that the PHC nurse has received the necessary training and development and that the latest evidence and research is accessed and used by the PHC nurse.
- Audit that training programmes and professional development opportunities are available and that they are accessed by the PHC nurse with support from the provider manager.

Managing chronic ill-health, high blood pressure and asthma

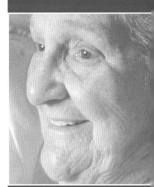

In this case scenario a man who had experienced chronic asthma and high blood pressure was assisted to live a more active life. Through long-term management the practice nurse was able to stabilise the client's symptoms and prevent complications of asthma and high blood pressure from occurring.

Health gain for client
Asthma and hypertension stable: client leads a more active life. Less time spent at hospital.
Target: *The Health of the Nation* Coronary Heart Disease (DoH 1992).

Quality health interactions with PHC nurse
The client's experiences
- *"If you're worried you can just walk in."* (Indicator 1)
- *"She never rushes me, she really listens and understands."* (Indicator 2)

- "I can go to the nurse about anything, she makes her assessment and calls the doctor if necessary." (Indicator 3)
- "She knows what she is talking about and talks to you in a language you can understand." (Indicator 4)
- "She knows me personally and knows my problems." (Indicator 5)
- "She listens to what I have to say and then we talk about what we can try." (Indicator 6)
- "I can talk to her about anything, she makes me feel comfortable." (Indicator 7)
- "Before at the hospital I used to see a different person every time and have to explain my history … the nurse knows me and my complaints." (Indicator 8)
- "The nurse acts on my behalf to get information from the hospital." (Indicator 9)
- "I was too breathless to get to the surgery to have my ulcers dressed so the nurse talked to the district nurse who then started to come in three times a week." (Indicator 10)

Goals and actions of PHC nurses
- *Promotion* of health through evidence-based management of asthma and hypertension.
- *Empowerment* of the client to cope and manage the asthma symptoms and to recognise when medical assistance is needed.
- *Enable* the client to adapt and cope with the symptoms and lead an active life.
- *Eliminate or reduce* the underlying causes of ill health e.g. environmental factors such as tobacco smoke and causes of hypertension.
- *Reduce* the impact of ill health experienced by the client by education about the causes and management techniques he can use.
- *Arrest or retard* the progress of degenerative health problems by symptom management.
- *Compensate* for the effects of his diseases and enable him to adapt.
- *Prevent* avoidable acute asthma attacks and complications of hypertension.
- *Identify* the effects of disease on the client's life.
- *Impact* on *Health of the Nation* Coronary Heart Disease (DoH 1992) targets by stabilising blood pressure to decrease the risk of stroke and heart disease.

Prerequisites
- A practice profile of health and disease patterns is used.
- The goals and strategy of care is long-term chronic disease management and prevention of deterioration through monitoring the client's health.
- There is sustained support from other staff members in the multidisciplinary team (MDT) which enables the PHC nurse to concentrate on the skilled task of chronic disease management.
- The role and function of members of the MDT is explicit and there is effective communication and liaison.
- There are regular practice team meetings to discuss case management and the services offered by the practice. There are attached health visitors and district nurses who work closely with the team.

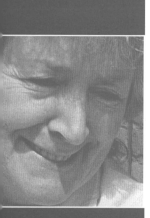

- Many of the patients in the practice are known individually to the practice nurse, leading to continuity and the opportunity to influence health behaviour and outcomes in the long term.
- The client case-notes and client feedback enable evaluation. This can be reviewed on an individual and practice level.
- The PHC nurse has received training and updates. The PHC nurse reviews journals etc. to keep up to date.

Auditing, measuring and monitoring quality

- Client feedback to confirm ease of accessibility to the PHC nurse, the nurse's approachability and that there was sufficient time with the PHC nurse. Client evaluation of the extent to which he was involved in goal setting and treatment planning. Was the care client-centred and non-judgmental? Feedback from the PHC nurse regarding the above and the ability of the PHC nurse to work with the multidisciplinary team.
- Client feedback concerning their perception of the efficacy of the advice and information given to the client.
- Audit the client-held and nursing/medical records for evidence of stability of blood pressure and asthma. Documentation of interprofessional collaboration and liaison.
- Audit the type of support staff available and what their roles are in relation to overall service delivery.
- Audit that the PHC nurse works to evidence-based and up-to-date protocols and guidelines.
- Monitor the number of clients seen during the clinic and the time taken with clients and compare it to other times and annual numerical returns.
- Does the practice have a chronic disease register?
- Check when the service is used most heavily.
- Audit the nature of client visits and contrast them to known local and national health needs.
- Audit that the PHC nurse has received the necessary training and development and that the latest evidence and research is accessed by the PHC nurse.
- Audit that training programmes and professional development opportunities are available and that they are accessed by the PHC nurse with support from the provider manager.

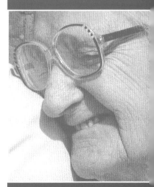

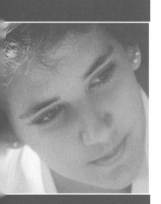

Sustaining breast-feeding post partum

In the following scenario the mother was struggling to continue to breast-feed. She had been at the point of giving up and starting to bottle feed when she received support and advice from the family health visitor at the ten day post-partum home visit.

Health gain for client

Sustained breast-feeding for over three months post-partum and adapting positively to parenthood.
Target: *The Health of the Nation* Mental Health (DoH 1992).

Quality health interactions with PHC nurse

A mother's experiences
- *"The health visitor came to visit me at home which was best for me because it was private."* (Indicator 1)
- *"She gave me the time that I needed."* (Indicator 2)
- *"She knew what my problems were."* (Indicator 3)
- *"The health visitor suggested ways which might help me to cope."* (Indicator 4)
- *"She took account of my family's individual circumstances."* (Indicator 5)
- *"I was so tired the health visitor recognised this."* (Indicator 6)
- *"She didn't criticise me for thinking about bottle-feeding or not coping well."* (Indicator 7)
- *"I was able to ring the health visitor or pop into the clinic if I needed advice."* (Indicator 8)
- *"I know that I can talk to her if I have any problems in the future."* (Indicator 9)
- *"There were other health visitors who knew me because they worked as a team."* (Indicator 10)

Goals and actions of PHC nurses

- *Promotion* of physical, cognitive, social and educational development of the baby by sustaining breast-feeding (Greene *et al.* 1995).
- *Empowerment* of client to breast-feed her child which is known to improve cognitive development (Greene *et al.* 1995) and reduce the risk of gastro-enteritis (Newman 1995).
- *Enable* individuals and communities to adapt and cope with life event, i.e. parenthood.
- *Eliminate or reduce* the anxiety of the parent in adapting to parenthood.
- *Reduce* the impact of ill health e.g. reduce the risk of post-natal depression and potential for gastro-enteritis by giving appropriate support (Beck 1995).
- *Arrest or retard* the effects of family stress and reduce the likelihood of postnatal depression.
- *Compensate* for the effects of a major life event i.e. parenthood, through giving support and advice.
- *Prevent* avoidable postnatal depression and early cessation of breast-feeding.
- *Identify* delayed physical, cognitive, and/or social development through regular monitoring and assessment.
- *Impact* on *Health of the Nation* Mental Health (DoH 1992) targets by identification of environmental and local causes of disease and ill health.

Prerequisites

- There is a balanced skill mix within the health visiting team to enable the PHC nurse to have time to support the mother to achieve her goal to breast-feed.
- The PHC nurse is able to work with other members of the PHC teams to offer consistent support.
- Most of the PHC nurse's time is spent with the client in her home environment where the client feels most relaxed.
- Data is available regarding local breast-feeding patterns and prevalence. A needs assessment is available to demonstrate the local need for support for first time parents and breast-feeding.
- The success of the intervention can be elicited from recorded interventions and outcomes in the client-held and PHC nurse-written records. Client feedback will elicit the satisfaction and influence that the PHC nurse service has offered.
- The PHC nurse is up to date with current research and works in accordance with Trust and national policies in infant feeding practices and has access to breast-feeding counsellors and support groups to offer to parents.

Auditing, measuring and monitoring quality

- Client feedback to confirm ease of access to the PHC nurse, approachability of the PHC nurse and that there was sufficient time with the PHC nurse. Client evaluation of the extent to which they were involved in goal setting and treatment planning. Was the care client-centred and non-judgmental? Feedback from the PHC nurse regarding the above and ability of the PHC nurse to work in a health promoting way.
- Client feedback concerning their perception of the efficacy of the advice and information given to them.
- Audit the client-held and nursing/medical records for evidence of sustained breast-feeding. Documentation of interprofessional collaboration, liaison and advocacy.
- Audit the type of support staff available and what their roles are in relation to overall service delivery.
- Audit that the PHC nurse works to evidence-based and up-to-date protocols and guidelines.
- Monitor the number of clients seen and the time taken with clients and compare it to other times and annual numerical returns.
- Check when and where the service is used most heavily.
- Audit the content of client visits and PHC nurse home visits and contrast them to known local and national health needs.
- Audit that the PHC nurse has received the necessary training and development and that the latest evidence and research is accessed by the PHC nurse.
- Audit that training programmes and professional development opportunities are available and that they are accessed by the PHC nurse with support from the provider manager.

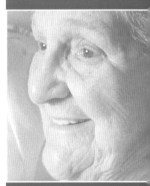

Supporting behaviour change management for parents whose child won't settle to sleep

The parents in the next case scenario attended a child health sleep clinic for three months. The clinic is run by a health visitor and child psychologist and forms part of an early intervention team set up to address child protection issues which are a recognised health need within the health authority area.

Health gain for clients

Sustained behaviour change in sleep patterns for a family with a young child who does not settle to sleep. Parents learn skills of behaviour modification which they are also now using to manage other aspects of childcare. Parents report that they are less stressed. Target: *The Health of the Nation* Mental Health (DoH 1992).

Quality health interactions with PHC nurse

Parents' experiences

- *"We quickly got an appointment which was great; we were at our wit's end."* (Indicator 1)
- *"They listened to our point of view."* (Indicator 2)
- *"They understood our difficulties."* (Indicator 3)
- *"They knew what they were doing; we learned to trust their advice."* (Indicator 4)
- *"They let us move at our own pace."* (Indicator 5)
- *"We decided what to do together; we chose the best option for us."* (Indicator 6)
- *"They didn't judge us if we didn't achieve the goals we'd set."* (Indicator 7) (Hewitt *et al.* 1996)
- *"It was helpful to see the same person each week."* (Indicator 8)
- *"It was our health visitor who made the referral and put us in touch with them."* (Indicator 9)
- *"They [the PHC nurse and psychologist] work together using their own special skills."* (Indicator 10)

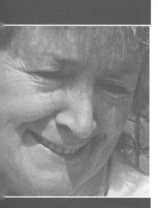

Goals and actions of PHC nurses

- *Promotion* of parental awareness of physical, cognitive, social and educational development of the child.
- *Empowerment* of parents to adapt their behaviour and identify ways to change behaviour patterns.
- *Enable* parents to adapt and cope with behavioural issues.
- *Eliminate or reduce* the underlying causes of the parents' anxieties.
- *Reduce* the impact of stress from the presenting problem.
- *Arrest or retard* the problems experienced by the parents.
- *Compensate* for the stresses of parenthood by helping the parents to identify management techniques.
- *Prevent* avoidable stress and anxiety for the parents and help them to feel more relaxed with parenting.
- *Impact* on *Health of the Nation* Mental Health (DoH 1992) targets by identification of behaviour change and coping techniques.

Prerequisites

- Goals and strategies are formulated by the PHC nurse and the psychologist. The goals and strategies are agreed with the clients and are reviewed at each visit. The service is client led. The PHC nurse works in partnership with the clients, and care is non-judgmental and client-centred.
- A district profile to determine the level of need for a sleep clinic.
- Support staff enable the PHC nurse to spend more time doing clinical work. Information about the early intervention service is available so that parents are aware of its potential.
- The PHC nurse works in partnership with the psychologist and each practitioner brings their own respective expertise to the intervention.
- The clinic environment is welcoming and comfortable seating in a private room is available. Clients choose their appointment time and the frequency of their visits.
- Evaluation is done by the client. Documentation of progress is kept by the client and the PHC nurse.
- The PHC nurse has access to up-to-date research and attends training and updates.

Auditing, measuring and monitoring quality

- Client feedback to confirm the speed and ease of accessibility to the PHC nurse, that the nurse was approachable and that there was sufficient time with the PHC nurse. Client evaluation of the extent to which they were involved in goal setting and treatment planning. Was the care client-centred and non-judgmental? Feedback from the PHC nurse regarding the above and ability of the PHC nurse to work in a health promoting way.
- Client feedback concerning their perception of the efficacy of the advice and information given to them.
- Audit the client-held and clinic records for evidence of behaviour change and sustained improvement. Documentation of interagency collaborations, i.e. with the family health visitor.
- Audit the type of support staff available and what their roles are in relation to overall service delivery.
- Audit that the PHC nurse works to evidence-based and up-to-date protocols and guidelines.
- Count the number of clients seen during the clinic and the time taken with clients and compare it to other times and annual numerical returns.
- Check when the service is used most heavily.
- Audit the nature of client visits and contrast them to known local and national health needs.
- Audit that the PHC nurse has received the necessary training and development and that the latest evidence and research is accessed by the PHC nurse.
- Audit that training programmes and professional development opportunities are available and that they are accessed by the PHC nurse with support from the provider manager.

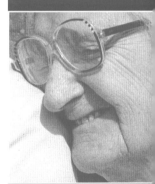

Preventing childhood accidents

The family seeking political asylum had been housed in a temporary first floor flat. The health visitor and the team are aware of the local prevalence of accidents to children in the Trust area and have recently set up a cost price accident equipment scheme available to families with low incomes. During an initial home visit the health visitor assessed that there was a risk of the children falling from the windows. The mother also asked for advice on buying a safety harness for the youngest child.

Health gain to client

The windows in the flat are locked and a safety harness is obtained and used.
Target: *The Health of the Nation* Accident prevention (DoH 1992).

Quality health interactions with PHC nurse

Mother's experiences
- *"By coming to my home the health visitor was able to see the dangers."* (Indicator 1)
- *"I was able to ask her how to get a safety harness."* (Indicator 2)
- *"The health visitor knew what the problems were."* (Indicator 3)
- *"She knew all about the dangers."* (Indicator 4)
- *"She really got to know me and what I felt."* (Indicator 5)
- *"I decided what I needed."* (Indicator 6)
- *"She didn't make me feel bad about not sorting out the windows earlier."* (Indicator 7)
- *"I can phone her or make an appointment at the surgery to see her when I need to."* (Indicator 8)
- *"The health visitor wrote to the housing association to ask them to fix the windows."* (Indicator 9)
- *"I've been put in touch with social services by the health visitor to get more help."* (Indicator 10)

Goals and actions of PHC nurses

- *Promotion* of parental awareness about risks to children from accidents.
- *Empowerment* of the parent to prevent accidents.
- *Enable* the parent to prevent accidents.
- *Eliminate or reduce* the underlying risk factors contributing to accidents.
- *Reduce* the impact of poor housing and the risk of accidents on busy local roads by promoting and providing safety equipment.
- *Arrest or retard* the risk of accidents.
- *Compensate* for the effects of unavoidable hazards.
- *Prevent* avoidable accidents.
- *Identify* potential risk factors in the context of normal child development.
- *Impact* on *Health of the Nation* Accident prevention (DoH 1992) targets by identification of environmental and local causes of accidents.

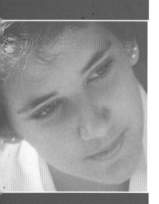

Prerequisites

- The philosophy of the Trust and the health authority is focused on evidence-based preventive working practices.
- Appropriate support staff are available.
- The PHC nurse works in partnership with other members of the multidisciplinary team and the local authority.
- Prevalence rates of childhood accidents are determined through the information flow from local accident and emergency departments.
- A health needs assessment has shown the local need to concentrate on accident prevention for children under five years of age.
- The venue for the contact is in the client's home where a thorough assessment of need can take place.
- Evaluation through PHC nurse documentation of the process and outcomes is available in the client and PHC nurse records.
- Staff are trained in the skilled assessment of accident prevention interventions.

Auditing, measuring and monitoring quality

- Client feedback to confirm ease of accessibility to the PHC nurse and that there was sufficient time with the PHC nurse. Client evaluation of the extent to which they were involved in goal setting and treatment planning. Was the care client-centred and non-judgmental? Feedback from the PHC nurse regarding the above and why a home visit is critical to successful outcomes. Client feedback can also elicit uptake and satisfaction with the service.
- Client feedback concerning their perception of the efficacy and acceptability of the advice and information given to the client.
- Audit of the client-held and nursing records for evidence of uptake of the service and compliance with advice and information given. Documentation of interagency collaboration with other professionals and agencies.
- Audit the type of support staff available and what their roles are in relation to overall service delivery.
- Audit that the PHC nurse works to evidence-based and up-to-date protocols and guidelines.
- Count the number of clients seen and the time taken with clients and compare it to other times and annual numerical returns.
- Assess the uptake of the accident prevention equipment scheme to demonstrate its popularity and value to clients.
- Audit the nature and content of PHC nurse home visits and contrast them to known local and national health needs and targets.
- Audit that the PHC nurse has received the necessary training and development and that the latest evidence and research is accessed by the PHC nurse.
- Audit that training programmes and professional development opportunities are available and that they are accessed by the PHC nurse with support from the provider manager.

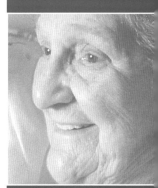

5

Performance management based on quality

A framework for monitoring the quality of primary health care nursing services

The empirical work underpinning this guide demonstrates a clear link between indicators of quality and outcome in terms of tangible health gain. However, the relationship between nursing 'inputs' and subsequent health 'outcomes' is still poorly understood although a movement towards effective measurement of the process using short-term or intermediate proxy indicators is gradually being achieved.

The indicators of quality and prerequisite checklist provide a framework for measuring and monitoring the process and outcome of PHC nursing interventions.

Templates for quality audit of primary health care nursing services, with suggestions for incorporating audit routes throughout the contracting process are described in this section. These templates represent an initial statement and provocation on the challenging issue of measuring quality and process. They require further refinement and development.

It is important to define the roles and contributions of each set of stakeholders in terms of data collection, action and audit. The responsibilities of commissioners, service providers and PHC nurses are clearly identified below with suggestions for approaches to strengthening contract specificity and possible audit routes. The final part of this section addresses the contribution of the client as consumer in the quality monitoring process. More detailed suggestions for questions that could be incorporated into a formal audit tool can be found in Appendix 3 (*see* p. 33).

The purchasing/commissioning role in quality performance management

Commissioners can play a key role in influencing the quality of PHC nursing through ensuring that an appropriate level of detail is incorporated into service specifications. They can exert further influence by making certain that the contracted services are informed by consumer and provider perspectives.

Failure to articulate expectations of quality in an explicit form will undermine the performance management process. This will have a particular impact on the ability of the provider managers and PHC nurses to deliver care which is effective and high quality. The indicators and prerequisite checklist provide useful pegs both for service specification and for subsequent audit and quality monitoring.

Suggested approaches to influencing quality at the commissioning level
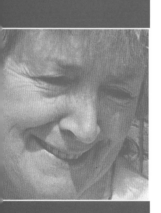
- ○ Ensure that contracted services are informed by 'grass roots' client and provider perspectives (Harding 1996).
- ○ Ensure that the contracts stipulate the expectation of designated roles and responsibilities for the PHC nurse within the MDT (King's Fund 1996).

- Set contract requirements which encourage a balanced skill and grade mix that will enable a PHC nurse specialist to carry out skilled client-related tasks (HVA 1994, Ross and MacKenzie 1996).
- Require evidence of demonstrable communication between staff e.g. MDT meetings where 'action points' are recorded.
- Require evidence of an annually reviewed and updated profile of locally defined health needs.
- Require providers to demonstrate active consumer involvement and the use of client-held records.
- Agree strategic objectives with providers of services and client representatives. Audit that the process indicators are being incorporated into practice development programmes e.g. the establishment of a practice charter (Ishmael and Duffy 1995, Greagsby 1996, Buck *et al.* 1997).
- Audit the use and review of evidence-based practice protocols, standards and guidelines which are used and reviewed by the MDT (Antrobus and Brown 1996).
- Require providers to use a range of audit tools to evaluate quality in PHC nursing services.

The organisational/service provider role in quality performance management

Provided that appropriate service specifications at the commissioning level are in place, those responsible for managing PHC nursing services can take steps at an organisational level to maximise the potential for health gain by putting in place a number of mechanisms. These will enable PHC nurses to incorporate the ten quality indicators into their practice.

Suggested approaches to influencing quality at the organisational/service provider level

Commissioners and providers of PHC nursing services can audit for quality in a number of ways:

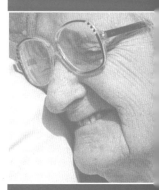

- Audit of the clinic environment: through both inspection and consultation with PHC staff and users. Examine the available facilities, e.g. private rooms for consultations and response times to client-led consultation requests (King's Fund 1996, DoH 1996a).
- Audit timings of PHC nurse clinics and time available for PHC nurses to visit clients at home. Ensure that services are appropriate to locally identified health needs and client-led needs (Roberts *et al.* 1996a).
- Audit for evidence that appropriately trained, registered specialised PHC nurses are responsible for needs assessment, care planning, evaluation and review of client health status (Ross and MacKenzie 1996).
- Audit for evidence that an annual review and update of health need profiles is undertaken and that this is a MDT collaborative exercise.
- Audit for evidence that a minimum annual level of training and professional development is offered to PHC nurses and that the content of the training meets health

needs assessments. This will include the training and development of staff in measuring and evaluating quality and effectiveness. Audit that records are kept to show that this has been achieved (Ross and MacKenzie 1996, DoH 1996a, King's Fund 1996).

- Audit uptake and fluctuations in service use in order to identify less efficient services and contract for changes in the service which meet local demand, e.g. less popular clinic sessions, or a low uptake in screening services (Roberts and Phipps 1996b).

The primary health care nurse's role in quality performance management

PHC nurse's involvement in the audit of their practice is currently largely confined to the monitoring of the number and type of contact. Practitioners have an important role to play in the evaluation of quality and effectiveness of their interventions. The prerequisite checklist and indicators provide a useful framework for this activity.

Suggested approaches to influencing quality at the PHC nursing level

- Audit client health records for evidence of identification of client-centred health goals and health-focused intervention plans.
- Audit client health records to ascertain that agreed treatment plans, evaluation of health benefits and appropriate follow-up, discharge and review by the PHC nurse has taken place (King's Fund 1996).
- Audit of the use of up-to-date evidence-based health needs protocols.
- Audit client health records including evidence of the processes which facilitate measurements of health improvements e.g. stable blood pressure, health behaviour changes over time and less need to seek medical and nursing intervention (Ishmael and Duffy 1995).

The client contribution in quality performance management

The importance of harnessing a consumer perspective in assessing quality is increasingly well recognised. Some ways in which clients' own experiences of the services can assist the audit processes are outlined below.

Suggested approaches to influencing quality at the consumer level

- Audit of the clients' experiences of health improvements and health behaviour change resulting from nurse–client interactions (Ross and MacKenzie 1996).
- Audit through questionnaires to clients about their satisfaction and perceptions of health 'wants and needs' (Cowpe et al. 1994, Rees Lewis 1994).
- Gain clients' views about their satisfaction with the service and its outcome.
- Utilise consumer research on health-related topics.
- By using client focus groups gather clients' opinions of services.
- Through information gathered by heads of quality in both Trusts and health authorities about quality in practice.
- Through monitoring complaints systems and information from them via GP practices, Trusts and health authority levels or via the community health councils.
- By incorporating the practice-based client participation groups.

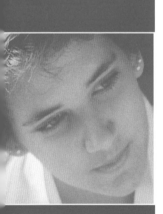

Outline of the project

Review of research literature to identify quality indicators using accident prevention as a model.

Series of focus group workshops with purchasers and providers to explore the relevance and usefulness of quality indicators: PHC nurses, PHC nurse managers, health promotion specialists, primary care commissioners, HA and GP purchasers.

Refined set of practice-based quality indicators generated, relating to PHC nurse input into accident prevention.

Indicators validated against existing research data.

Wider literature review of research on indicators and quality in PHC nursing.

Exploratory work
Series of interviews with PHC nurses from different disciplines looking at quality issues.

Series of information gathering interviews with purchasers: HA and GP purchasers to elicit the usefulness and degree of need for quality indicators.

Identification of six case-study sites health visitors (n=4), practice nurses (n=2).

Case-studies
Observation of the processes of client–PHC nurse interactions (n=24) followed by reflective interviews with clients and the PHC nurse to determine their view of quality elements and health gain in each interaction.

Analysis of data from case-studies
- Insights gained into the client's perception of quality PHC nursing and consequent health benefits/gain.
- List of indicators leading to health improvements generated.
- Clear view of infrastructure identified: opportunities and barriers influencing the ability of PHC nurses in putting indicators into practice. Checklist of prerequisites generated.
- Processes leading to health improvement/benefits identified.
- Evidence of intermediate health benefits identified.
- Formulated ways to monitor and commission refined set of practice-based quality indicators related to the PHC nurse-client interaction which had a health benefit.

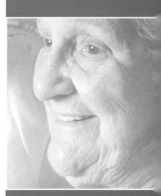

How the indicators of quality impact on health benefits

The process	Indicators of quality
Nurse–client interaction	*The setting*

The process — Nurse–client interaction:

- Client meets nurse in appropriate venue.
- Client does not feel rushed and can raise health needs.
- Nurse listens and understands.
- Nurse applies expertise and knowledge.
- Appropriate advice and information given to client by nurse.
- Client makes choices and decisions with nurse. Plan of care devised.

Indicators of quality — The setting:

- Choice and ease of access to PHC nurse.
- Time with PHC nurse.
- Skilled and accurate identification of health needs.
- PHC nurse is an informed practitioner who advocates and works in collaboration with other agencies and groups.
- PHC nurse is credible to client. Individualised approach. Non-judgmental.
- Partnership approach using client-centred agenda.

Continuity of care ensures long-term benefits maintained.

HEALTH BENEFIT DERIVED BY CLIENT

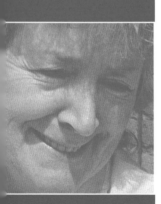

Suggested focus for formal audit tool questions based on quality indicators and the prerequisite checklist

To be completed by provider managers/administrators

- What is the average uptake for the clinics in terms of numbers?
- Are some clinics over-subscribed or under-subscribed?
- Do the type of clinics available reflect the health needs profile of the locality?
- What provision is made to learn about local needs from a client viewpoint?
- Does the training and development which staff attend reflect local and national health strategies?
- Do staff meet regularly in the locality?
- What other means of communication have been identified within the organisation?

To be completed by primary health care nurses

- Are the process and outcomes of the assessment, planning and outcome/evaluation documented in client-health records? Does this include evidence of client involvement in determining health needs and goals?
- What do the client records show about health benefits being achieved in the short, intermediate and long term?
- What are the nurse's views on the skill/grade mix balance within the team and where are the gaps in service (if any)?
- Are practice guidelines and protocols used? When were they last updated?
- Is there a locally based practice profile of health issues available? When was it last updated and who contributed to it?
- Is the nurse's practice based on the latest knowledge base (evidence-based)?
- What professional training and development has the nurse attended in the last year?
- How frequently does the nurse meet formally and informally with other members of the PHC team?

To be completed by the client

- Are the clinics convenient, friendly and accessible? (choice and accessibility of services)
- Is there enough time to talk about what is important? (sufficient time)
- Was the advice/information given to you relevant? (skilled assessment)
- Was the advice given by the nurse appropriate and did the nurse appear to understand the issues? (informed and credible practitioner)
- Did the information or advice given to you make a difference? (individualised approach)
- Who determined what was discussed and what could be achieved? (client-centred partnership approach)
- Did you feel that the nurse made assumptions about what you needed without checking your thoughts and wishes? (non-judgmental approach)
- Have you seen the same member(s) of the nursing team on a regular basis? (continuity of care)
- Has the nurse represented your views and needs to others on your behalf? (advocate for clients)
- Does the nurse work with or know other people involved in your care? (liaison and collaboration with other professionals and agencies)

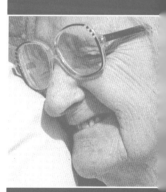

References

Antrobus, S. and Brown, S. (1996) 'Guidelines and protocols: a chance to take the lead', *Nursing Times*. vol. 92, no. 23, pp. 38 – 9.

Antrobus, S. and Brown, S. (1997) 'The impact of the commissioning agenda upon nursing practice: a proactive approach to influencing health policy', *Journal of Advanced Nursing*. vol. 25, pp. 309 – 15.

Appleby, F. (1991) 'In pursuit of excellence', *Health Visitor*. vol. 64, no. 8, pp. 254 – 6.

Barić, L. and Barić, L. (1995) *Health promotion and health education*. Barns Publications, Hale Barnes, p.152.

Beck, C.T. (1995) 'Perceptions of nurses' caring by mothers experiencing postpartum depression', *JOGNN*. November/December, pp. 819 – 25.

Billings, J.R. and Cowley, S. (1995) 'Approaches to community needs assessment: a literature review', *Journal of Advanced Nursing*. vol. 22, pp. 197 – 301.

Brown, P.A. and Piper, S. M. (1997) 'Nursing and the health of the nation: schism or symbiosis?', *Journal of Advanced Nursing*. vol. 25, pp. 197 – 301.

Buck, D., Godfrey, C. and Morgan, A. (1997) 'The contribution of health promotion to meeting health targets: questions of measurements, attribution and responsibility', *Health Promotion International*. vol. 12, no. 3 (forthcoming).

Cowley, S. (1993) 'Skill mix: value for whom?', *Health Visitor*. vol. 66, no. 5, pp. 166 – 71.

Cowley, S. (1996) 'Achieving positive outcomes: principles and process', *Health Visitor*. vol. 69, no. 1, pp. 17 – 19.

Cowpe, M., Maclachlan, A. and Baxter, E. (1994) 'Clients' views of a health visiting service', *Health Visitor*. vol. 67, no. 11, pp 390 – 1.

Crown, L. (1996) 'Community information systems: getting it right this time', *Health Visitor*. vol. 69, no. 2., pp. 68 – 70.

Dahl, R. (1995) 'Creating the environment necessary to ensure quality patient care in the community setting', *Seminars for Nurse Managers*. vol. 3, no. 3, pp. 146 – 51.

Dines, A. and Cribb, A. (1993) *Health promotion: concepts and practice*. Blackwell Scientific Publications, Oxford.

DoH (1992) *The Health of the Nation a consultative document for health in England*. DoH, London.

DoH (1993) *Targeting practice: the contribution of nurses, midwives and health visitors to The Health of the Nation*. DoH, London.

DoH (1996a) *The National Health Service – a service with ambitions*. DoH, London.

DoH (1996b) *Primary care: the future*. NHS Executive.

DoH (1996c) *Executive Letter (96) 94*. NHS Executive.

DoH (1997) 'Public health in England strategy speech' (Unpublished). Tessa Jowell, MP, Minister of State for Public Health, London.

Donabedin, A. (1992) 'The role of outcomes in quality assessment and assurance', *Quality Review Bulletin*. November, pp. 356 – 60.

Family Heart Study Group (1994) 'Randomised control trial evaluating cardiovascular screening in intervention in general practice: principal results of British Family Heart Study', *British Medical Journal*. vol. 308, pp. 313 – 20.

Gibbins, R.L., Riley, M. and Brimble, P. (1993) 'Effectiveness of programme for reducing cardiovascular risk for men in one general practice', *British Medical Journal*. vol. 306, pp. 1652 – 6.

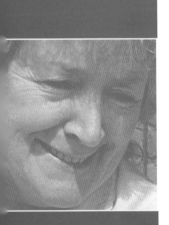

Gillespie, R. (1996) 'Meeting targets', *Journal of Community Nursing.* vol. 10, no. 6, pp. 8 – 10.

Gillis, A. (1995) 'Exploring nursing outcomes for health promotion', *Nursing Forum.* vol. 30, no. 2, pp. 5 – 12.

Greagsby, P. (1996) 'Life preservers', *Health Service Journal.* 4 July, pp. 28 – 9.

Greene, L.C., Lucas, A., Livingstone, M.B.E., Erasmus, P.S., Harland, G., Baker and Brian, A. (1995) 'Relationship between early diet and subsequent cognitive performance during adolescence,' *Biochemical Society Transactions.* vol. 23, p. 376s.

Griffiths, P. (1995) 'Progress in measuring nursing outcomes', *Journal of Advanced Nursing.* vol. 21, pp. 1092 – 1100.

Harding, M. (1996) 'So what do community nurses do?' *Health Service Journal.* 11 April, pp. 26 – 7.

Hewitt, K., Heatherley, S. and Ibrahim, J. (1996) 'Are pre-bedtime routines necessary?' *Health Visitor.* vol. 69, no. 5, pp. 181 – 3.

HVA (1994) *Action for health: an HVA guide marketing skill mix campaigning.* HVA, London.

Imperial Cancer Research Fund OXCHECK Study Group (1994) 'Effectiveness of health checks conducted in primary health care: results of the OXCHECK study after one year', *British Medical Journal.* vol. 308, pp. 308 – 12.

Ishmael, N. and Duffy, T. (1995) 'Health visitor outcomes – an effective model', *Value for Money Update.* vol. 1, pp. 14 – 15.

Jeffreys, L.A., Clark, A.L. and Koperski, M. (1995) 'Practice nurses' workload and consultation patterns', *British Journal of General Practice.* vol. 45, no. 397, pp. 415 – 18.

Kendrick, D. (1994) 'Role of primary health care team in preventing accidents to children', *British Journal of General Practice.* vol. 44, no. 385, pp. 372 – 5.

King, W. (1995) 'Counting what counts', based on the speech given to the 1994 HVA Annual Professional Conference 20-22 October, in Torquay. *Health Visitor.* vol. 68, no. 1, pp. 14 – 15.

King's Fund (1996) *King's Fund organisational audit: primary health care organisational standards and criteria.* King's Fund, London.

Kitson, A.L., Harvey, G. and Guzinska, M. (1988) *Nursing quality assurance direction* 2nd edition. RCN Standards of Care Project, Royal College of Nursing and King's Fund, London.

Laidman, P. (1987) *The role of the health visitor in the prevention of accidents to children.* Child Accident Prevention Trust with the HEA, London.

Latter, S., Macleod Clark, J., Wilson-Barnett, J. and Maben, J. (1992) 'Health education in nursing: perceptions of practice in acute settings'. *Journal of Advanced Nursing.* vol. 17, no. 1, pp. 164 – 72.

Luker, K.A. (1990) 'Gaining access to clients: the case of health visiting'. *Journal of Advanced Nursing.* vol. 15, no. 1, pp. 74 – 82.

Macleod Clark, J., Wilson-Barnett, J., Latter, S. and Maben, J. (1992) 'Health education and health promotion in nursing: a study of practice in acute areas'. Unpublished Research Report, Department of Health.

Macleod Clark, J. (1993) 'From sick nursing to health nursing' in Wilson-Barnett, J. and Macleod Clark, J. (Eds.) *Research in Health Promotion and Nursing.* The Macmillan Press Ltd, London.

McMurray, A. (1992) 'Expertise in community health nursing', *Journal of Community Health Nursing.* vol. 9, no. 2, pp. 65 – 75.

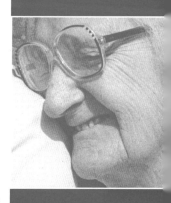

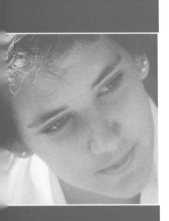

Mant, J. and Hicks, N.R. (1996) 'Assessing quality of care: what are the implications of the potential lack of sensitivity of outcome measures to differences in quality?' *Journal of Evaluation in Clinical Practice.* vol. 2, no. 4, pp. 243 – 8.

Newman, J. (1995) 'How breast milk protects newborns', *Scientific American.* December, pp. 58 – 61.

Peckham, S and Spanton, J. (1994) 'Community development approaches to health needs assessment', *Health Visitor.* vol. 67, no. 4, pp. 124 – 5.

Redfern, S. J. and Norman, I. J. (1994) *The validity of quality assessment instruments in nursing: final report to Department of Health.* Nursing Research Unit, King's College, London.

Rees Lewis, J. (1994) 'Patient views on quality care in general practice: literature review', *Social Science and Medicine.* vol. 39, no. 5, pp. 655 – 670.

Roberts, I., Kramer, M. and Suissa, S. (1996a) 'Does home visiting prevent childhood injury? A systematic review of randomised control trials'. *British Medical Journal.* vol. 312, pp. 29 – 33.

Roberts, C. and Phipps, J. (1996b) 'Setting up an out-of-hours child health clinic', *Health Visitor.* vol. 69, no. 2, pp. 72 – 3.

Ross, F. and Mackenzie, A. (1996) *Nursing in primary health care: policy into practice.* Routledge, London.

Rourke, A.M. (1991) 'Self-care: chore or challenge?' *Journal of Advanced Nursing.* vol. 16, no. 2, pp. 233 – 41.

Savage, J. (1995) *Nursing intimacy an ethnographical approach to nurse-patient interaction.* Scutari Press, Trowbridge.

Simnett, I. (1995) *Managing health promotion developing healthy organisations and communities.* John Wiley & Sons, Chichester.

Stretcher, V.J., Bauman, K.E., Boat, B., Glen Fowler, M., Greenberg, R. and Stedman, H. (1993) 'The role of outcome and efficacy in an intervention designed to reduce infants' exposure to environmental tobacco smoke'. *Health Education Research.* vol. 8, no. 1, pp. 137 – 43.

Summers, A. and McKeown, K. (1996) 'Health needs assessment in primary care: a role for health visitors', *Health Visitor.* vol. 69, no. 8, pp. 323 – 4.

Timpka, T., Svensson, B. and Molin, B. (1996) 'Development of community nursing: analysis of the central services and practice dilemmas', *International Journal of Nursing Studies.* vol. 33, no. 3, pp. 297 – 308.

Twaddle, S., Liao, X.H. and Fyvie, H. (1993) 'An evaluation of postnatal care individualised to the needs of the woman', *Midwifery.* vol. 9, no. 3, pp. 154 – 60.

WHO (1985) *Targets for Health for All: targets in support of the European regional strategy for Health for All by the Year 2000.* WHO Regional Office for Europe, Copenhagen.

The ten indicators of quality in PHC nursing

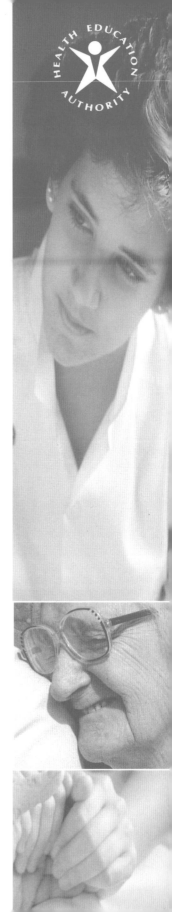

1	Choice of services and accessibility of service to client
2	Sufficient time
3	Skilled assessment of health needs
4	Informed and credible practitioner
5	Individualised approach
6	Client-centred partnership approach
7	Non-judgmental approach
8	Continuity of care
9	Acting as an advocate for the client
10	Liaison and collaboration with other professionals and agencies

Processes through which health benefits are achieved

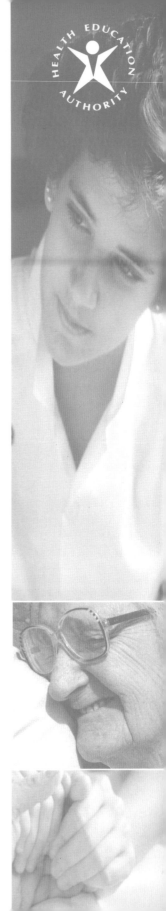

A case scenario template

Health gain for client
- Tangible improvements in health status, well-being and quality of life.
- Coping, adapting and changes in knowledge or behaviour pertinent to health status.

Quality health interactions with PHC nurse
- The influence of the ten process indicators on quality interactions.

Goals and actions of PHC nurses
- Promotion of physical, cognitive, social and educational development.
- Empowerment of clients, families and communities to prevent disease and minimise existing ill health.
- Enable individuals and communities to adapt and cope with life events.
- Eliminate or reduce the underlying causes of disease rather than treating the resulting ill health.
- Reduce the impact of ill health.
- Arrest or retard the progress of chronic health problems.
- Compensating for the effects of life events.
- Prevent avoidable accidents/incidents.
- Identify delayed physical, cognitive or social milestones.
- Impact on *Health of the Nation* (DoH 1992) targets by identification of individual, environmental and local causes of disease and ill health to maximise potential for health and well-being.

Prerequisites
- The structural and organisational elements which give the opportunity for quality characteristics to be incorporated into PHC nursing practice.

Auditing, measuring and monitoring quality
- The purchasing and auditing framework which drives the process.

Adapted from Ishmael and Duffy (1995).

Prerequisites for quality: a checklist

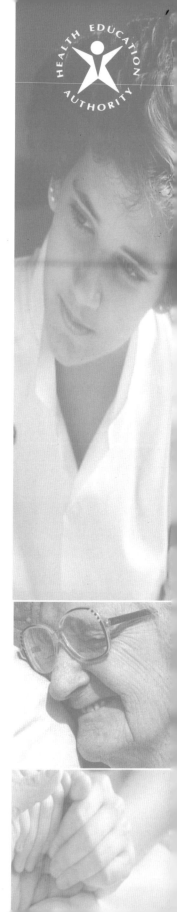

Explicit HP goals and strategies for PHC nursing interactions
- Are goals explicitly stated and are they embedded in principles of preventive care?
- Are goals articulated in terms of the achievement of measurable short-, medium- and long-term health benefits?
- Do goals and strategies move beyond crisis management, the achievement of contact targets and national policy outcomes? (Brown and Piper 1997, Buck *et al.* 1997)

Partnership approach
- Do clients hold their own records?
- Are clients involved in defining their own health goals and making decisions?
- Are clients involved in service needs identification and evaluation processes?

Appropriate skill mix
- Does the skill/grade mix provide adequate numbers of highly skilled PHC nurses to undertake adequate assessment and complex interventions? (Jeffreys *et al.* 1995, Cowley 1993)
- Is the skill/grade appropriate to meet the health needs of the population?
- Are support staff trained to an appropriate level?

Integrated team work
- Does the MDT demonstrate clear structures and roles, MDT care planning, communication mechanisms and collaborative networks and information technology systems such as e-mail? (King's Fund 1996, Ross and MacKenzie 1996, Antrobus and Brown 1997)

Appropriate environment and flexibility
- Is there choice in terms of venue and out-of-hours services for PHC nursing input including home- and community-based visiting depending on client need?
- Is the clinic environment user-friendly and accessible to all groups of consumers? (King's Fund 1996, Roberts *et al.* 1996b).

Profile of health needs
- Are PHC nursing-planned interactions defined by locally identified population health needs profiling? (Peckham and Spanton 1994, Billings and Cowley 1995, Summers and McKeown 1996)
- Are shared databases utilised to ensure collaboration and reduce duplication? (Ross and MacKenzie 1996)

continued overleaf

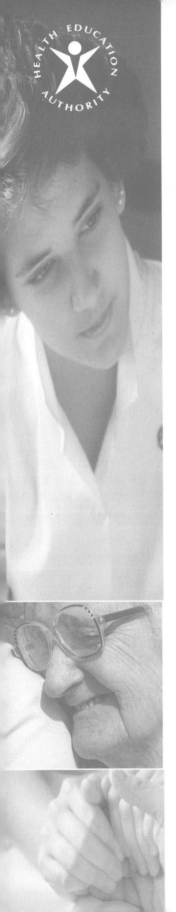

Appropriate evaluation strategy

○ Are providers using a range of audit and measurement tools to evaluate the quality of their services? (Mant and Hicks 1996, King's Fund 1996)

Practice development strategy

○ Are providers demonstrating active investment in PHC nursing staff through access to further education, libraries and current research?
○ Does this include skills updating and specialist training?
○ Are practice guidelines and protocols continually updated to reflect new research evidence? (Antrobus and Brown 1996, 1997)

How the indicators of quality impact on health benefits

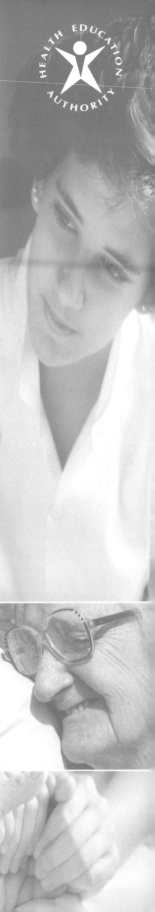

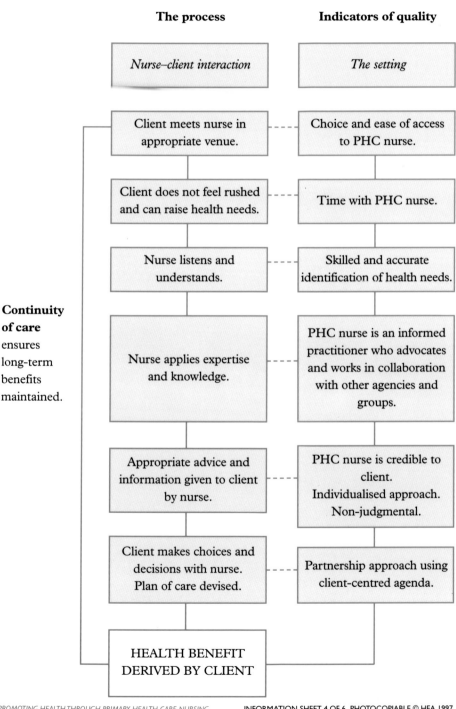

The process	Indicators of quality
Nurse–client interaction	*The setting*
Client meets nurse in appropriate venue.	Choice and ease of access to PHC nurse.
Client does not feel rushed and can raise health needs.	Time with PHC nurse.
Nurse listens and understands.	Skilled and accurate identification of health needs.
Nurse applies expertise and knowledge.	PHC nurse is an informed practitioner who advocates and works in collaboration with other agencies and groups.
Appropriate advice and information given to client by nurse.	PHC nurse is credible to client. Individualised approach. Non-judgmental.
Client makes choices and decisions with nurse. Plan of care devised.	Partnership approach using client-centred agenda.

Continuity of care ensures long-term benefits maintained.

HEALTH BENEFIT DERIVED BY CLIENT

Suggested focus for formal audit tool questions

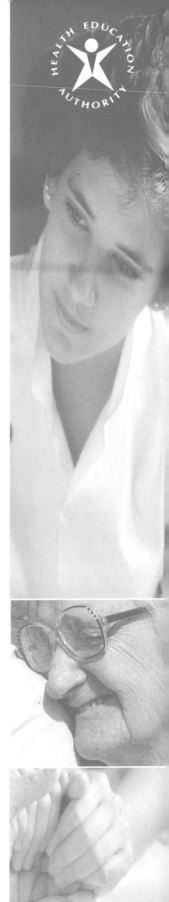

To be completed by provider managers/administrators
- What is the average uptake for the clinics in terms of numbers?
- Are some clinics over-subscribed or under-subscribed?
- Do the type of clinics available reflect the health needs profile of the locality?
- What provision is made to learn about local needs from a client viewpoint?
- Does the training and development which staff attend reflect local and national health strategies?
- Do staff meet regularly in the locality?
- What other means of communication have been identified within the organisation?

To be completed by primary health care nurses
- Are the process and outcomes of the assessment, planning and outcome/evaluation documented in client-health records? Does this include evidence of client involvement in determining health needs and goals?
- What do the client records show about health benefits being achieved in the short, intermediate and long term?
- What are the nurse's views on the skill/grade mix balance within the team and where are the gaps in service (if any)?
- Are practice guidelines and protocols used? When were they last updated?
- Is there a locally based practice profile of health issues available? When was it last updated and who contributed to it?
- Is the nurse's practice based on the latest knowledge base (evidence-based)?
- What professional training and development has the nurse attended in the last year?
- How frequently does the nurse meet formally and informally with other members of the PHC team?

To be completed by the client
- Are the clinics convenient, friendly and accessible? (choice and accessibility of services)
- Is there enough time to talk about what is important? (sufficient time)
- Was the advice/information given to you relevant? (skilled assessment)
- Was the advice given by the nurse appropriate and did the nurse appear to understand the issues? (informed and credible practitioner)
- Did the information or advice given to you make a difference? (individualised approach)
- Who determined what was discussed and what could be achieved? (client-centred partnership approach)
- Did you feel that the nurse made assumptions about what you needed without checking your thoughts and wishes? (non-judgmental approach)
- Have you seen the same member(s) of the nursing team on a regular basis? (continuity of care)
- Has the nurse represented your views and needs to others on your behalf? (advocate for clients)
- Does the nurse work with or know other people involved in your care? (liaison and collaboration with other professionals and agencies)

A framework for monitoring the quality of primary health care nursing services

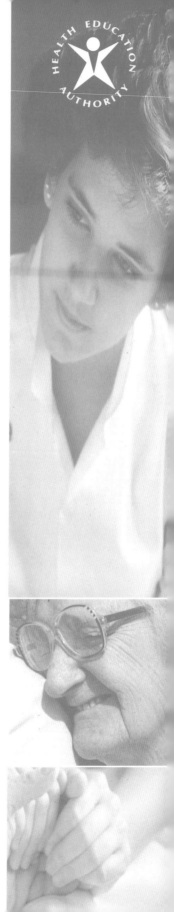

Suggested approaches to influencing quality at the commissioning level

- Ensure that contracted services are informed by 'grass roots' client and provider perspectives (Harding 1996).
- Ensure that the contracts stipulate the expectation of designated roles and responsibilities for the PHC nurse within the MDT (King's Fund 1996).
- Set contract requirements which encourage a balanced skill and grade mix that will enable a PHC nurse specialist to carry out skilled client-related tasks (HVA 1994, Ross and MacKenzie 1996).
- Require evidence of demonstrable communication between staff e.g. MDT meetings where 'action points' are recorded.
- Require evidence of an annually reviewed and updated profile of locally defined health needs.
- Require providers to demonstrate active consumer involvement and the use of client-held records.
- Agree strategic objectives with providers of services and client representatives. Audit that the process indicators are being incorporated into practice development programmes e.g. the establishment of a practice charter (Ishmael and Duffy 1995, Greagsby 1996, Buck et al. 1997).
- Audit the use and review of evidence-based practice protocols, standards and guidelines which are used and reviewed by the MDT (Antrobus and Brown 1996).
- Require providers to use a range of audit tools to evaluate quality in PHC nursing services.

Suggested approaches to influencing quality at the organisational/service provider level

- Audit of the clinic environment: through both inspection and consultation with PHC staff and users. Examine the available facilities, e.g. private rooms for consultations and response times to client-led consultation requests (King's Fund 1996, DoH 1996a).
- Audit timings of PHC nurse clinics and time available for PHC nurses to visit clients at home. Ensure that services are appropriate to locally identified health needs and client-led needs (Roberts et al. 1996a).
- Audit for evidence that appropriately trained, registered specialised PHC nurses are responsible for needs assessment, care planning, evaluation and review of client health status (Ross and MacKenzie 1996).
- Audit for evidence that an annual review and update of health need profiles is undertaken and that this is a MDT collaborative exercise.

continued overleaf

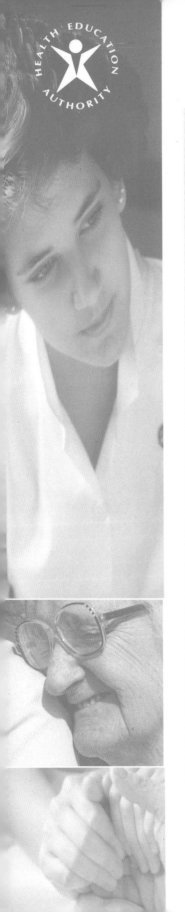

- ○ Audit for evidence that a minimum annual level of training and professional development is offered to PHC nurses and that the content of the training meets health needs assessments. This will include the training and development of staff in measuring and evaluating quality and effectiveness. Audit that records are kept to show that this has been achieved (Ross and MacKenzie 1996, DoH 1996a, King's Fund 1996).
- ○ Audit uptake and fluctuations in service use in order to identify less efficient services and contract for changes in the service which meet local demand, e.g. less popular clinic sessions, or a low uptake in screening services (Roberts and Phipps 1996b).

Suggested approaches to influencing quality at the PHC nursing level

- ○ Audit client health records for evidence of identification of client-centred health goals and health-focused intervention plans.
- ○ Audit client health records to ascertain that agreed treatment plans, evaluation of health benefits and appropriate follow-up, discharge and review by the PHC nurse has taken place (King's Fund 1996).
- ○ Audit of the use of up-to-date evidence-based health needs protocols.
- ○ Audit client health records including evidence of the processes which facilitate measurements of health improvements e.g. stable blood pressure, health behaviour changes over time; and less need to seek medical and nursing intervention (Ishmael and Duffy 1995).

Suggested approaches to influencing quality at the consumer level

- ○ Audit of the clients' experiences of health improvements and health behaviour change resulting from nurse–client interactions (Ross and MacKenzie 1996).
- ○ Audit through questionnaires to clients about their satisfaction and perceptions of health 'wants and needs' (Cowpe *et al.* 1994, Rees Lewis 1994).
- ○ Gain clients' views about their satisfaction with the service and its outcome.
- ○ Utilise consumer research on health-related topics.
- ○ By using client focus groups gather clients' opinions of services.
- ○ Through information gathered by heads of quality in both Trusts and health authorities about quality in practice.
- ○ Through monitoring complaints systems and information from them via GP practices, Trusts and health authority levels or via the community health councils.
- ○ By incorporating the practice-based client participation groups.